Hotel/Motel Workout:

A Healthy Exercise Guide when Living on the Road

Copyright 2015 by Vernon R. Payne

ISBN-13: 978-1542879538

DEDICATED TO

MY MOTHER SOFIA

Acknowledgements

Let me first thank my family for encouraging me to write this book years ago, when we would talk endlessly during our summer vacations about things we wanted to do one day.

I want to thank those people who gave me the assistance I needed to complete the book. These include: the Hotel Director from Caserta, Italy, Francesco Lanzante; my cousin's husband Claudio Nottola, who arranged to let us shoot photos at the Hotel Europa; my cousin's daughter Livia, an accomplished ballerina and dancer, who posed for many of the exercise photos while we were in Italy.

Special thanks to Machelle Collins, the Day Manager of the Hampton Inn Suites in Columbus, Ohio, who let us photoshoot in one of the suites at the hotel. Also my colleague Molly Linek, who posed for the majority of my exercise photos. My son Chris also lent his time and body for the endeavor, as well as one of my good friends Lynn Morgan. Stan Deibert helped with the photoshoot and Edie Buckle helped with typing and editing.

I also want to recognize Molly's husband Scott, who helped me with this project as a copyright attorney.

Last but not least, thanks to my wife of 40 years, Cindy, for assisting me with photoshoots, editing and acting as a sounding board when I needed one.

About the Author

Vernon Rosendo Payne has a Bachelor of Science degree in Education from The Ohio State University and has been involved in the exercise industry for over 25 years. Aside from his individual weight-lifting routines, he coached high school football and tennis, which led him to work with youth for weight training, muscle gain and endurance to be applied to their specific sport.

After retiring from teaching high school, he continued to coach football while pursuing a personal training certification. He began to work at the local YMCA and not only earned YMCA training certification, but also acquired ACE (American Council of Exercise) certification. This allows him to train individuals both in and outside the YMCA.

He has attended a multitude of training clinics and seminars which address how to deal with metabolic syndrome (people at risk for diabetes, high BP, high blood sugar and coronary heart disease). He has studied and incorporates the methods of Rest-Based Training, Interval Training, Youth Training and a multitude of techniques to build muscle and core stability.

At the YMCA, he has provided guidance and support to people at all levels of fitness and created training programs for individuals and groups. He continues to train young people as well as older adults in strength and cardio conditioning.

Outside the Y, Vern also does personal training for people that don't go to an exercise facility or might not be able to leave their homes. As a certified personal trainer for over 10 years, he finds passion in what he does. He says that the passion for personal training is more important than the money at his age.

He enjoys hiking and is also an avid race walker, qualifying for the National Senior Olympics in 2015 by placing second at the regional finals in the 1500 meter and 5,000 meter events for his age group.

His wife and he have traveled extensively throughout North America and Europe.

His philosophy in life is to think young and stay fit as long as possible in order to enjoy life and its possibilities.

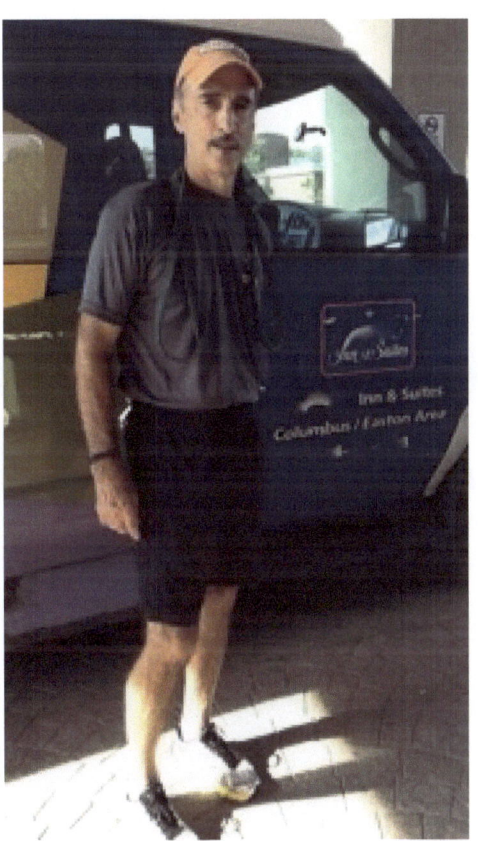

Table of Contents

NOTES

Chapter One

Hotel/Motel Workout Plan

The Hotel/Motel Workout Plan is designed for those people who travel frequently and want a condensed exercise program that meets their busy and hectic schedules.

After many years of traveling and staying at various hotels and motels for my job, I have come to the conclusion that most people would like to do some form of exercise while they are away from home and not be stuck watching TV and going out to eat during their free time. Folks like to have an exercise routine when they are at home and would like to maintain a routine while away on business or vacation.

True, there are workout facilities in many hotels; however, these usually include a few treadmills and a handful of dumbbells. There is always outside running or walking if the weather is decent and you're in a safe neighborhood, but this can be limiting.

This is why I have envisioned the Hotel/Motel Workout Plan for people that are either obligated to travel or just plain like to do so. Years ago I used to carry exercise springs and light dumbbells in my car when I traveled out of town; now I carry a couple of exercise bands and use my body weight to do all my exercises. I'm a competitive race walker and love walking as exercise, which is not always possible.

I always feel out of sorts if I don't do something physical, so I decided it would be helpful if I could share these ideas and routines with others. In the following pages, you will find different types of exercises, photos, routines and hopefully motivation to work out when you are away from home.

Equipment:

In fact, you don't even need equipment when you use body-weight-only type exercises. In the following pages, I will give you exercises that can be done with bands or body weight only, so that you can travel light and still feel like you got a heck of a workout.

I used to bring two to four long metal springs that fit on the end of handles to do some of my workouts when traveling, which was very cumbersome. After a while, exercise bands (super bands/mini bands), made out of a rubber alloy came along, and I find them very light and easy to fit in my luggage, especially on a long trip or even overseas (SPRI super bands).

Note: you might also carry along an extra pair of shorts and a t-shirt or two with your sneakers, of course.

Timing:

Timing is important when planning a workout. If you're on a business trip, you should plan for early morning before breakfast or any meetings that are scheduled. If you do a 30-minute routine, make sure you drink a glass of water before you start. After a shower and breakfast, you can make it to that first meeting by 9:00 a.m. fresh and ready to go. The other alternative is to wait until your day's meetings and work are finished and before you set out for dinner. You can come back to the room, change into your workout clothes, do your 30-45 minute routine, shower and head out to dinner feeling less stress with a healthy appetite (after you have burned 300 to 400 calories).

If you're really health conscious, you can exercise twice every day during the work week; I will give you a 5-Day program to follow later in the book.

Vacations might be a little different since you're normally out of your regular habits and are probably on the go most of the day. This could be a good time to either do an early morning workout before the family wakes up, or just incorporate exercise into the day's activities.

Remember, walking is one of the best exercises we can do and vacations usually involve some walking. Walking can relieve stress, keep your blood pressure down, keep your legs toned, lower your resting heart rate, and can be a very social thing to do.

Nutrition:

I'm not going to mention a lot about nutrition because that is not my expertise; however, what you put into your mouth is the most important thing you can do for a healthy body. This means when you eat out, look for the most nutritious food on the menu and how it is cooked. Try to stay clear of foods that are cooked with too much salt and fat. Don't be afraid to say how you want your food cooked; for example, baked is normally better than fried. Remember, fluid intake is just as important as your food choices so drink plenty of water, especially after a workout.

The timing of your meals is important in relation to your workout. Try not to exercise on a full stomach; always wait at least an hour after your meal to work out. In the morning, if you need to eat something before a workout, make it minimal and wait at least 1/2 hour before any physical activity.

I take my vitamins with some type of juice or water first thing in the morning and don't eat breakfast until after my workout. This way, I can get my needed proteins and carbs in to repair the muscle fibers that I tear down during the exercise. Lately, I have been taking a spoonful of coconut oil before a workout because it is processed quickly through the liver to provide quick energy, and doesn't settle in the fat tissue of the abdomen. A quick way to get that muscle recovery of carbs and proteins after a workout is to eat a bagel with peanut butter or drink a glass of some type of chocolate milk, but you can find the foods that work best for you.

The last thing I will mention is probably the most important; get a routine physical exam and discuss with your doctor what level of intensity or exercises you should attempt.

Remember that all exercise is good for the body, but there are some moves or intensities that may aggravate certain conditions. Your doctor may suggest modifications to some exercises. Be safe and have fun.

Chapter Two

The Structure of a Workout

In most of my exercise routines, I incorporate cardio and strength training in one package. You can also concentrate on strength only or cardio only on certain days. I will try to make this clear as I discuss the various components of the routines.

As an example, for instance, say you want to work on strength only one day; you might do a set of push-ups, then wait 30 seconds and do another set; then do a set of squats, wait 30 seconds and do another set. Your heart rate will increase but not to the level of a cardio workout. You might be, according to industry standards, at a zone one or two.

Now, you take those same two exercises and add a jump during your squat (jump squats) and only rest 10 seconds after your push-ups; then you've added a cardio element which, according to industry standards, puts you at a zone 2 or maybe even a zone 3 heart rate. Remember, the basic rule of thumb when it comes to cardio output is the talk test. In zone 1 (light intensity), you can carry on a conversation; zone 2 (moderate intensity), you're breathing harder, but you should still be able to talk; in zone 3 (high intensity), you might be able to say a few words, but you're mainly concentrating on your breathing; at zone 4, you're at your maximum heart rate and can only sustain this for a short period of time; an example would be the finish of a 100-meter dash.

I don't want to get too detailed in this book, because I know from experience that most of us want a simplified routine that can easily be remembered, and we don't have to spend hours reading about the human body and how exercise affects it. You have enough on your plate with your business or having fun with the family.

Structure of a workout:

I. **Warm-up** (*Dynamic Stretch*):

This constitutes dynamic movement of your muscles and joints. Some examples could be Jogging in place with knees high, High Kicks (Frankensteins), Butt Kicks, Arm Circles, reaching with arms to the sky or to the floor, or Squats. These are especially important when doing strength or intense body exercises. If you just want to walk fast, jog or run, you can start warming up by walking slowly and progressing to the stage you want to be in.

II. **Strength:**

Upper body - This could include Push-ups for the chest, back, triceps and core, with band work for the biceps, shoulders or back.

Lower body - This might include Squats, Toe Raises, Step-ups as well as using bands for Straight-leg Dead Lifts (Romanian Dead Lifts, also known as RDL's)

III. **Core:**

I like to list this as a separate category, even though you will be using your core in just about all the exercise that I recommend. Some of the more common core exercises include: Abdominal Crunches, Sit-ups, Supine Leg Lifts (on your back), Bird Dogs (on all fours with opposite leg and arm up), Supine Hip Extensions (bridge), Russian Twists (sitting with body leaning back, moving an object from side to side), Supermans (lying prone and extending arms and legs in an up and down movement), and Planks (push-up position or putting elbows on the floor).

IV. **Stretching**:

I usually recommend Static Stretches at the end of any routine, holding stretches without movement (no bouncing) for 20 to 30 seconds, because the muscles are warm and this allows for easy stretches and less risk of injury.

This is the basic structure of my workouts, but you can vary what you want to accomplish on a certain day; for example, you might not want to do your upper body two days in a row, or you just might want to do core exercises during a workout. I will recommend different routines, but you have flexibility in any workout. You can also vary your exercises during the same day or on different days. You may want to concentrate on cardio one day and strength on another. You can do strength in the morning and cardio in the evening. The choice is yours.

Chapter Three

The Beginner's Workout

Many individuals have never utilized an exercise program or have never exercised in a routine manner. So I am putting together a routine/ program that can be used by anyone, but especially those that feel intimidated or have never really tried to do a systematic exercise routine. This also includes my couch-potato friends.

The first thing that novices should realize is that they do not have to go to another room or workout area to exercise. They can achieve their goals and work up a sweat without leaving the room. The room itself will have articles and fixtures to utilize in a workout. For example, a chair can be used for Tricep Dips, a bed for Push-ups, or a book for Toe Raises.

Novice Workout (20 minutes)

Warm-up:

Stand, perhaps watching your favorite morning show; then walk in place, lifting your knees waist high (45 sec.); next, kick your feet high, keeping your legs straight (Frankensteins), (45 sec.); next, step side to side, pushing off on the outside foot as you come back to the middle (45 sec.); then use your arms to do small circles forward and backward, progressing to larger circles using the same motion (45 sec); lastly, point your hand to the sky, the other on your waist and then alternate hands, do the same out to each side, and then follow by bending down and pointing your hand to your foot, then alternate. You can say reach high, reach in the middle and reach low (45 sec.).

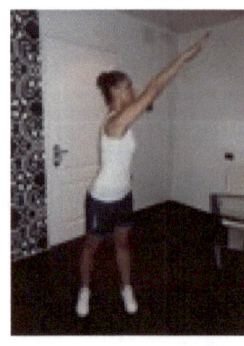 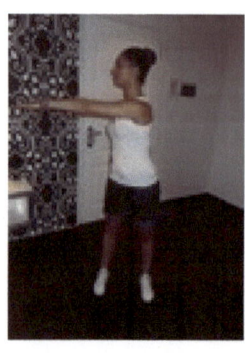 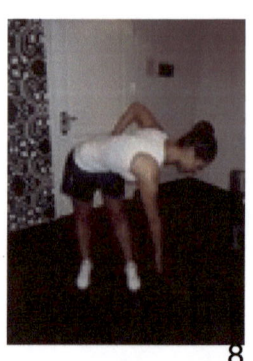

Strength:

Now that you're warmed up, you can start by doing some upper body exercises. In this case, you may use the bed for stability. Start by doing an elevated push-up at the side of the bed. Stand upright, then drop to the bed; with your chest about 2 inches from the mattress, push up. If this is too difficult, go to your knees before leaning on the bed and push up from there. Do 8 to 10 if you can, then stop to rest 20-30 seconds and repeat. Do 2 sets of 8 to 10 total, then rest for one minute. You can also do these by standing, leaning and pushing against the wall.

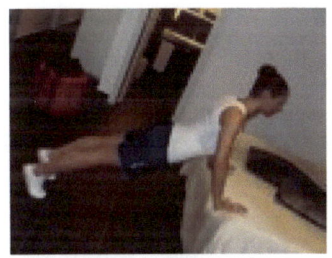

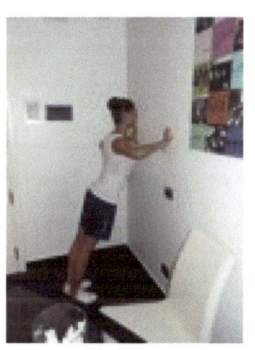

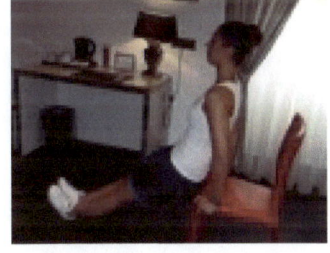 If the chair in the room has arms, you can do Tricep Dips. In a seated position, push yourself up, then set yourself down slowly. Again, do this 8 to 10 (reps) for 2 sets, again, rest for 20-30 sec. between sets. You can use a chair with no arms as shown in the picture, or if no appropriate chair is available, use the dresser or go to the floor, sitting with your hands behind you, feet flat on the floor. Lift one leg with hips off the floor and push up and come down with the elbows bent, repeat by pushing up again.

After resting a minute, you can work on the lower body, starting with what are called Prayer Squats. Set your feet a little wider than shoulder width apart, hinge your hips (get your buttocks pushed back), tighten/engage the abdominal muscles and keep your back straight, fold your hands in front of you, then slowly squat down, watching that your knees do not protrude over your toes. Then come up and repeat. Do 8 to 10 reps for 2 sets, rest 20 to 30 seconds between each set.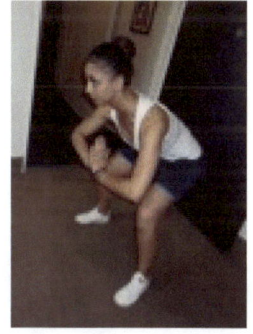

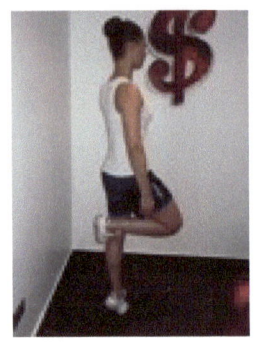

Next, let's try Toe Raises. If there is a book available, stand on the balls of your feet at the edge of the book, with your hands on the wall for support, and do 15 to 20 raises, 2 sets. For more intensity, try with one foot for 15 reps, then alternate.

Core:

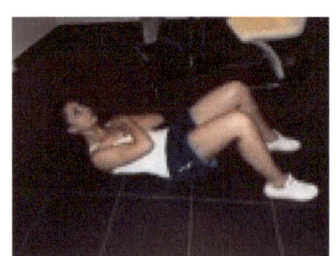

These can be done on the floor or on the bed. First let's start with the Crunch. Put your hands across your chest, knees up, feet flat on the floor or bed. Keep your eyes on the ceiling and lift your shoulders off the surface and hold for a count of 3, then go back down. Do 20 to 30 reps, stop, rest for 20-30 sec., then repeat.

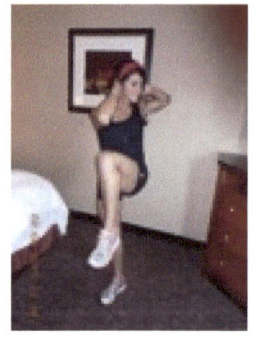

Another good core exercise is the Steam Engine. Stand, watching your favorite program again, with hands behind your head, elbows out. Now bend and lift your knee at the same time and touch the knee with the opposite elbow, now alternate. Count to 10, rest and do another set.

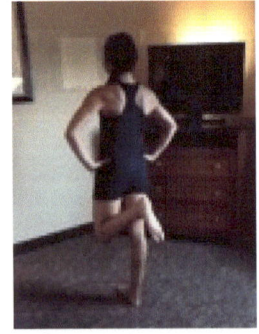

After you have finished with this exercise, try standing on one foot, either without touching or holding onto an object or hold on if you have to, for 30 seconds, then switch feet. You can extend the time for a progression.

Stretch :

Here you can do static stretches (no bouncing). These are easy movements that you hold for 20-30 seconds.

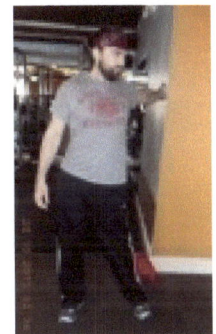

First, for a pectoral stretch, put your hand on the door jam, extend your arm, then turn your head in the opposite direction of the hand. Switch after 20-30 seconds.

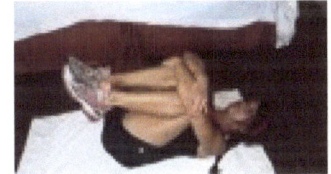

Next, lie flat, bring your knees up to your chest and hold 20-30 seconds; it's a great back stretch.

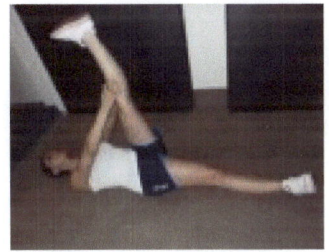

Then do a hamstring stretch either lying down on your back, one leg flat and the other at a 90-degree angle with both hands pulling from behind the calf of the raised leg, or in a standing position putting your leg up on the bed, keeping it straight while sliding your opposite hand down the shin to the ankle. If possible, hold for 20-30 seconds, then alternate legs.

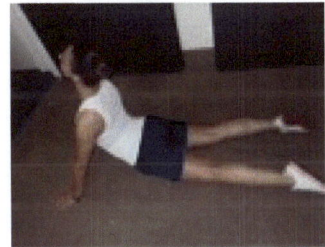

Finally, lie on the floor in a prone position (stomach), put your hands under the shoulders and push up (Cobra Move), hold for 20-30 seconds.

Now take a quick shower and have some breakfast before you head to that first meeting of the day.

Chapter Four

Body Weight 30x30

Body Weight 30X30 (30 minute program): This is a good all-around routine for those who don't carry exercise bands but want a quick routine before they head off for the day.

Warm-up: (Dynamic Stretch)

Make a little room you watch the begin by doing with a twist. Lunge sure your knees your toes, and twist then left while 10-12 reps. 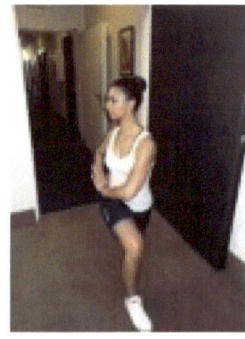 for yourself while morning news and forward lunges forward, making don't extend past your torso first right alternating legs.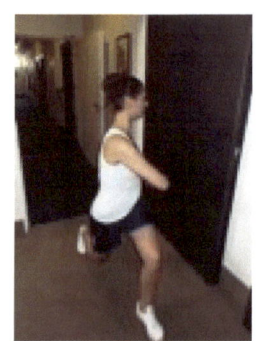

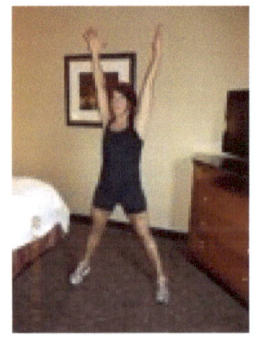 Next do a set of 10-12 jumping jacks, then do a set of Frankensteins, 10-12 reps where you kick your legs straight out and up, alternating.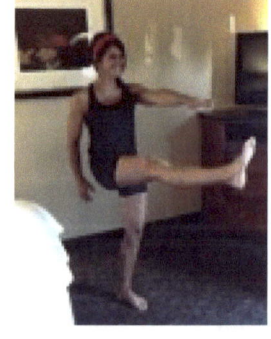

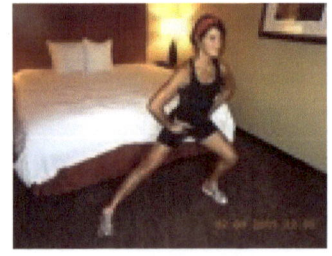 Next do lateral lunges, first lunging to the right, pushing back to the starting position, then repeat to the left. 10 reps on each leg.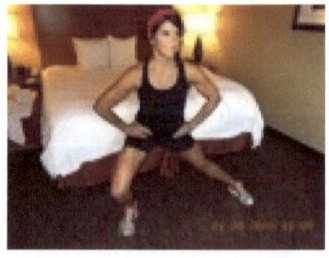

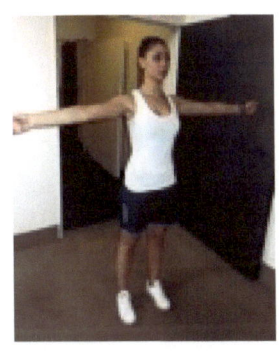

Last, get the arms moving in tight circles backward and forward for 30 seconds; then reach your right hand across your body above your head, then your left hand in the

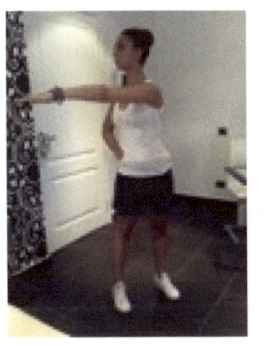

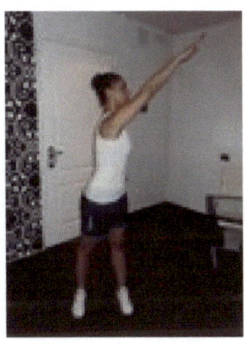

opposite direction. Repeat this at the midsection and then to the area below the knee; do several.

Strength and Cardio:

Since time is important when you're on the road and traveling, you can time each exercise. We'll start with 30 second work to 30 second rest (30X30). If you feel you need to progress and need more intensity, just up the work time and shorten the rest periods.

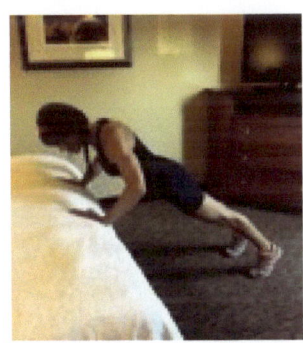

Push-ups (can be done on the floor or from the bed in an incline position). Do 2 sets of 30 sec. work and 30 sec. rest.

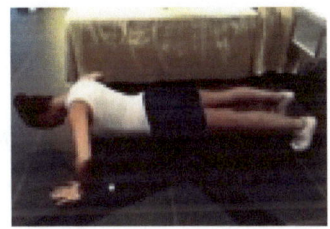

Tricep dips (You can use a desk, chair or bottom board of bed). You can also use the floor with hands behind you, one knee up and the other leg held off the floor. Again, it is 30X30, 2 sets.

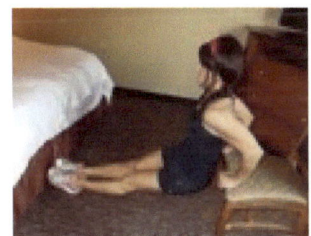

1/2 Burpee (A Full Burpee requires a push-up but with the 1/2, you put both hands down in front of you, kick back with both feet into a push-up position, then bring your feet back under your hips and jump up). 30X30, 2 sets

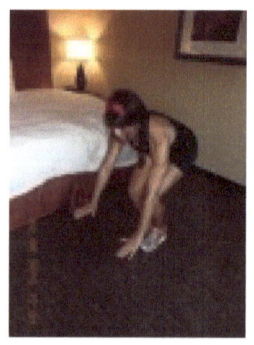 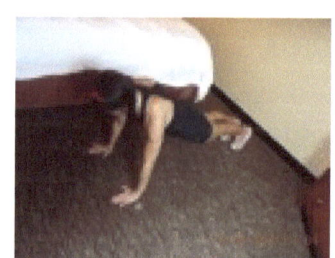 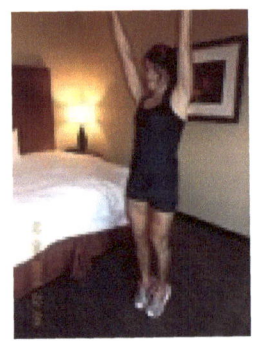

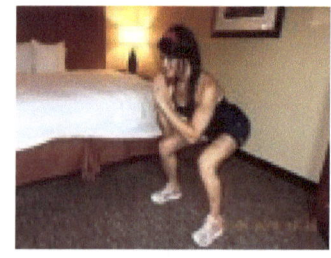

Prayer Squats (With hands folded in front, squat down tightening the abs. Push your glutes back, keeping your back straight. No knees over the toes). 2 sets of 30X30

Mt. Climbers (With hands on the floor in front of you and feet back in a push-up position, move your feet quickly in a climbing manner for 30 sec. then rest for 30). Do 2 sets

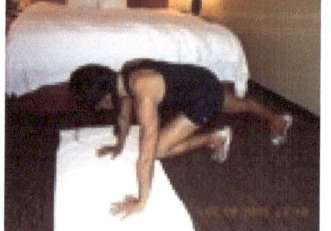 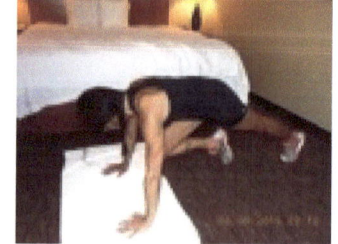

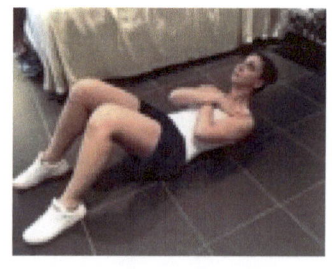

Crunches (In a supine position with hands across your chest and knees up, bring the shoulders off the ground and hold for 2 seconds). 2 sets of 30X30

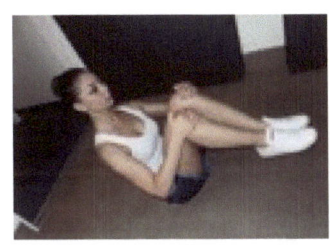 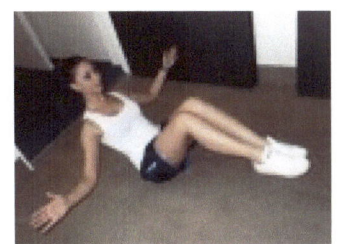

Ab Flies (In a seated position, lean back, kick your feet out with your arms outstretched, then bring your knees back towards your chest and bring the arms back to touch the knees). Work for 30 sec. and rest for 30 sec., then repeat.

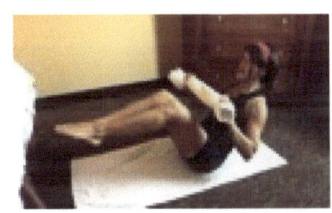 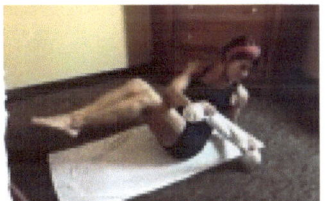

Russian Twist (In a seated position, lean back with a book or object in your hands and twist to the left, back to the middle, bringing the object up above your head. Then twist to the right and repeat back to the middle. 30X30 2 sets

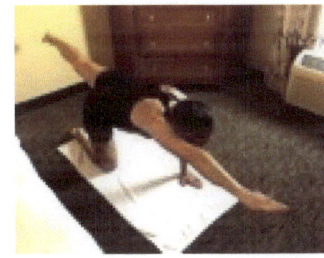

Bird Dog (Position yourself on all fours, then extend the right arm and left leg so that your back is level enough to hold a glass of water; now alternate right arm and left leg, hold each pose for 3 to 5 seconds. 30X30 2 sets

Stretch: (Hold each stretch for 20 to 30 seconds)

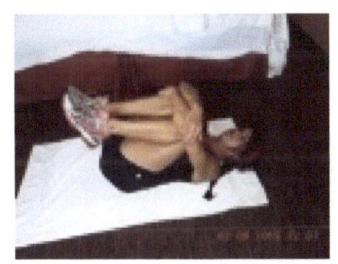

Bring your knees to your chest while lying on your back, hold. (**Lower Back Stretch**)

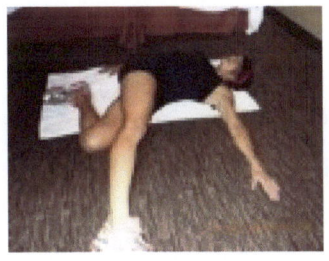

Drop your feet flat on the floor, drop your knees together to the left, keeping your shoulders flat, bring your right leg over the left knee and hold, repeat on the other side. (**Torso Stretch**)

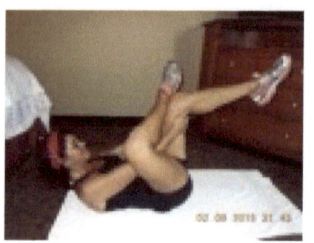

Put your left ankle over your right knee; with your hands under the right knee, pull toward you and hold; repeat on the other side (**P*iriformis* Stretch**).

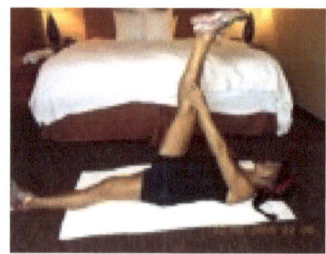

Now drop your left leg straight out flat and bring your right leg up in the air; grab behind the calf and hold, then repeat on the other side. (**Hamstring Stretch**)

Stand up and bring your hands down to the floor without bending your knees, (yoga) **Downward Dog**, trying to keep the heels down while you stretch your Achilles tendon and hold.

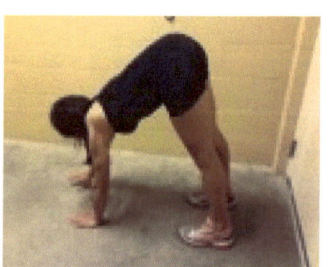

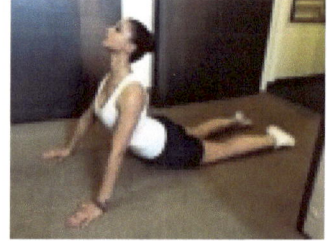

Finally, drop down with your hands under the shoulders and push up into a cobra (yoga) position and hold. (**Back Stretch**)

You should be ready for all activities and functions today. Just remember to eat a decent breakfast with protein and good carbs to build and rejuvenate those muscle cells.

Don't forget that you can also do this routine after you get back to the room from the day's work or play and before you eat dinner. If you're out of town for an extended period, you might do your exercise routine one day and do a 30-minute walk on another day. Or, if you're trying to stay in top condition for an athletic event of some kind, you can do an exercise routine in the morning and go for a run in the afternoon of the same day. You can always switch it up, depending on your schedule any day.

Chapter Five

Intense Workout Routine

I call this intense workout my Dirty Dozen, because I use 12 exercises that require an increase in cardio output. The amount of rest between the different exercises will keep you in either a Zone 2 or 3 heart level.

This routine is for the those hard-core workout junkies that require a little more sweat and feeling of accomplishment. It doesn't mean the average person who enjoys working out can't keep up; it just refers to the speed of the routine.

You can start the routine by working for 30 seconds and then taking a 30-second rest between exercises, which will still give you a pretty good sweat. You can vary the rest periods to your liking and you can always start out easy with a longer rest break, and decrease that rest the more you feel comfortable with the routine.

Modification of the exercises in the workout is important if you feel uncomfortable or if they hurt a particular joint and cause pain. You can modify any exercise either by going slower, walking to a position instead of jumping, or starting in an easier position such as beginning on your knees while doing a push-up instead of your toes.

You should be able to complete this routine in approximately 30 minutes or less. This does not include the warm-up or static stretch at the end. If you feel you need more endurance training, do 2 sets of both groups.

I. **Warm-Up**:

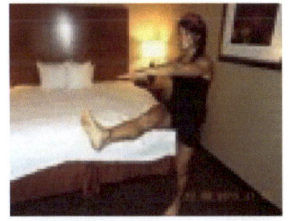

Basically you just want to move the major muscle groups of your body (Dynamic Stretch). Get the legs moving, straight leg kicks (Frankensteins), easy squats, lunges, arm movement in circles and overhead reaches to the right and to the left, or just jogging in place for a minute or two. A 5 to 10-minute warm-up is sufficient to get the juices flowing.

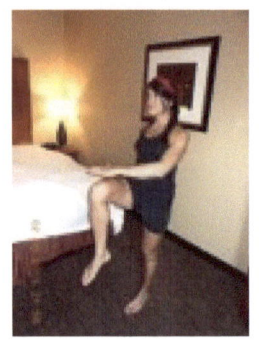 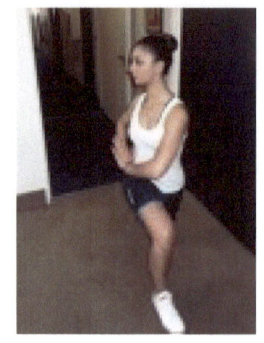 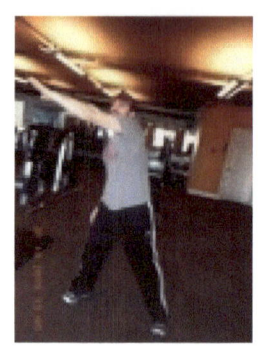 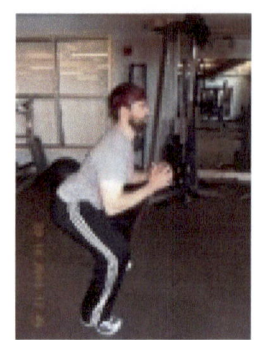

II. **Dirty Dozen 1**:

Strength/Cardio (30 seconds of work and 15/30 seconds rest) or (40 seconds of work and 15 seconds rest). Rest 1 minute between dozens.

Jumping Jacks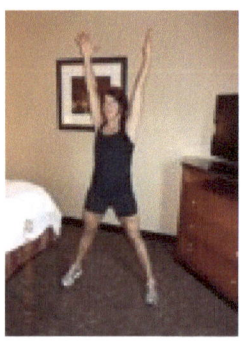

Lunge Jumps (switch legs in air)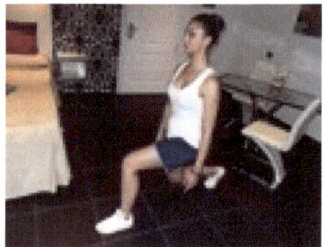

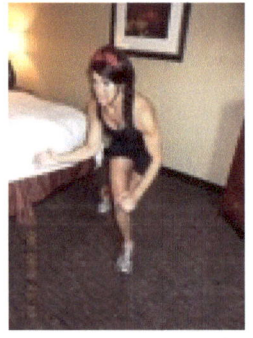 Ice Skaters (simulate motion)

Posterior Lunges (lunge behind)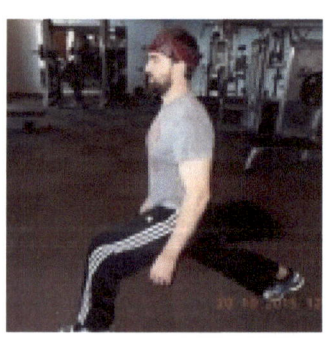

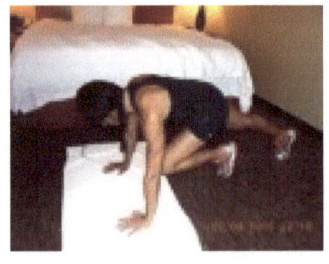 Mt.Climbers (move your feet back and forth)

Power Squats (jump up and land in a squat position)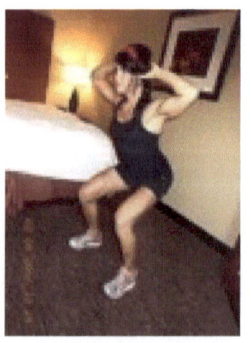

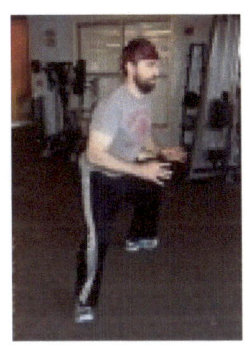

Frog Jump
(jump forward)

Frog Squats
(move upper
body down
and up)

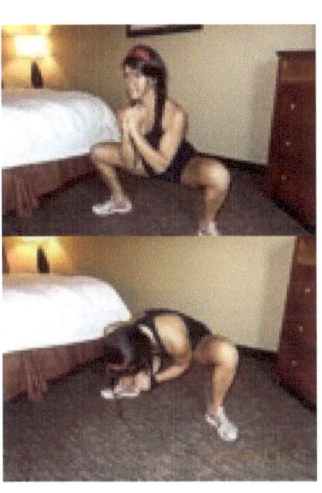

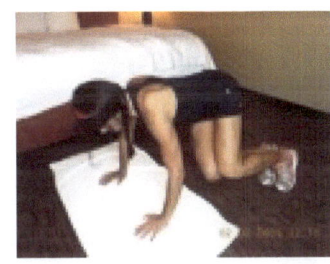

Moguls (feet together, jump side to side)

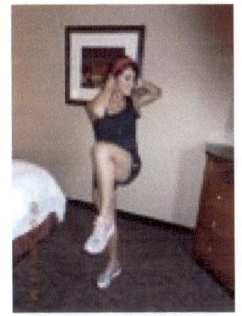 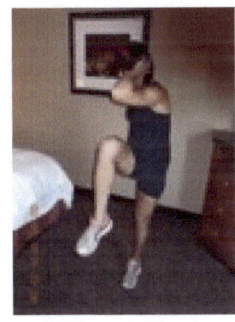

Steam Engine

Burpee

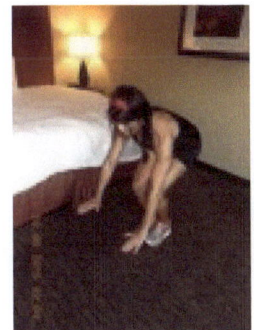 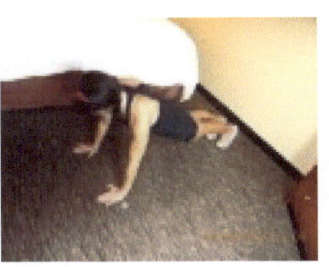 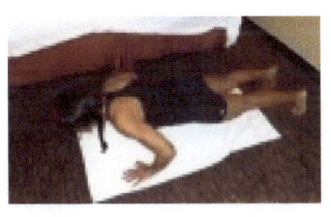 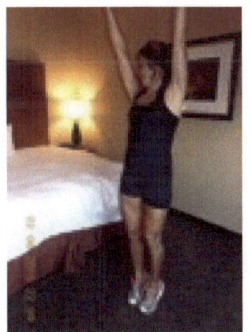

Prayer Squat

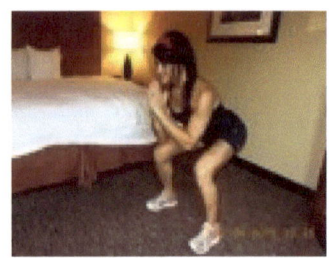

III. **Dirty Dozen 2**:

Cardio/Core (30 sec. work and 15/30 sec. rest) or (40 second work and 15 second rest)

Push-up   Oblique twist or V-up (elbow to knee)

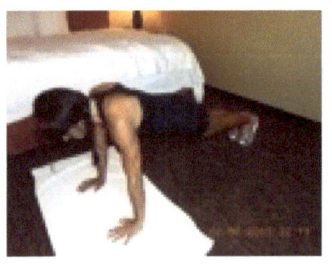   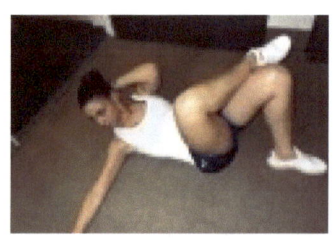   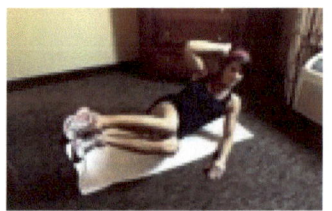

R e v e r s e
Crunches   Crunches

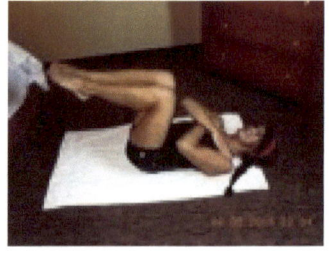

Scissors   Plank

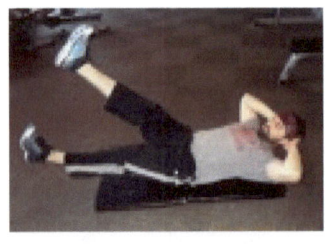   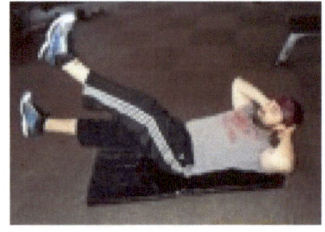   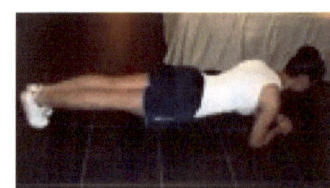

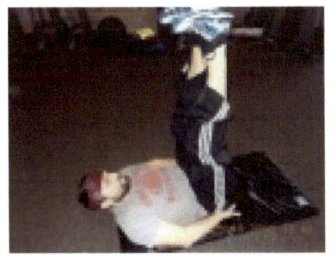

Hip Thrust
(keep legs up,
while thrusting
upwards)

Bird Dog

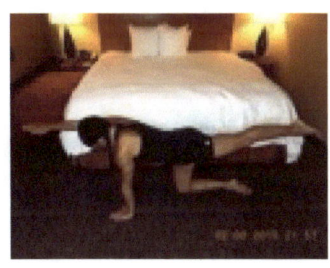

Russian Twist
(rotate to both
sides)

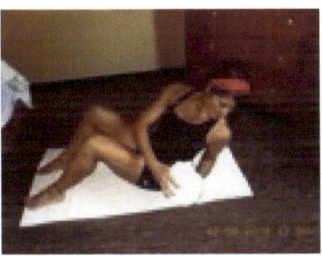

Superman
(hands and
feet up, hold,
then down)

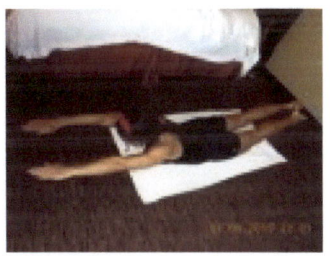

Bicycle Twist (rotate)

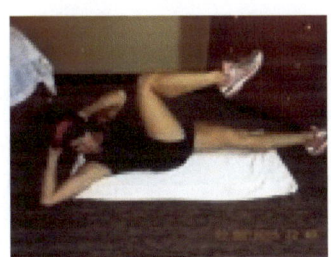

Ab Flies

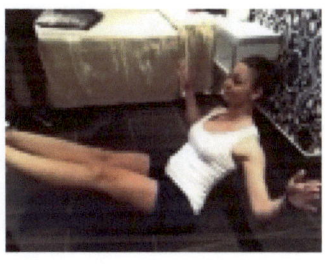

IV. **Stretch**:

Static Stretch, especially the main muscle groups. Hold each stretch
20 to 30 seconds.

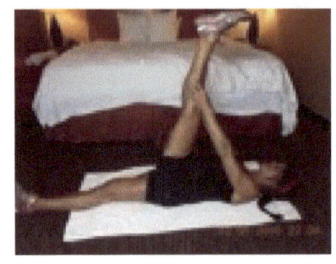

Hamstring

Piriformis

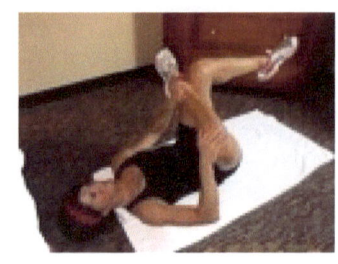

Butterfly

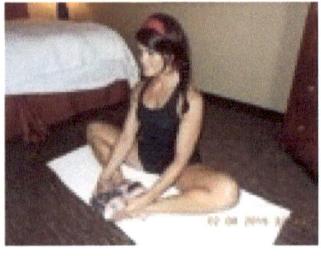

Achilles
Tendon

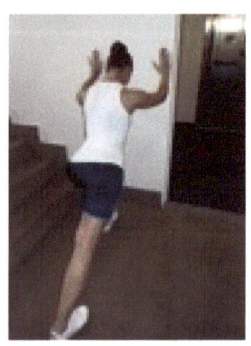

Cobra

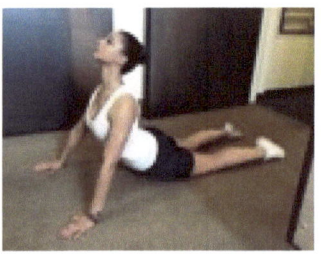

Downward
Dog

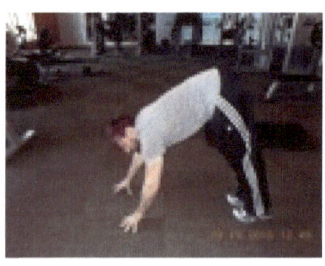

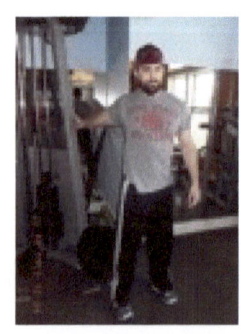

Pectorals

Lower Back

Chapter Six

Metabolic Workout/Burning Fat

It is obvious that in order to lose weight, we must lessen our intake of food, and studies have shown that 65 to 80 percent of weight loss depends on dietary changes. In this program, I will concentrate on the remaining 20 to 35 percent for successful weight loss by exercising.

According to dietary guidelines, most meals call for eating 20% protein, 25% fat and 55% carbohydrates, and most of us eat somewhere between 1,500 and 2,000 calories a day. But in order to lose one pound of body weight per week, you need either to eat 3,500 calories less or burn 3,500 calories more during that time. The more practical way to lose is through a combination of dietary changes **and** exercise. The important thing to remember when losing weight is that **you want to lose body fat and not muscle,** another reason to exercise.

I will leave the dietary component of any weight loss to a qualified nutritionist, and will focus on the exercise portion of burning fat and losing weight while maintaining a healthy body mass.

Burning more fat as we work out is something most of us desire to do. One of the best ways to do this is to increase the intensity of our routine for a short period of time, then lower the intensity for a longer period of time. Trainers refer to this as **high intensity interval training** or **HIIT** for short. A good example of this might be to find a high school track, then proceed to run the straight-aways and walk the curves. This could be a great 30-minute workout. This type of intensity variation allows our cells to get fired up and to burn fat for anywhere from 12 to 24 hours after a workout.

You can take any of the exercises I have discussed so far and increase the intensity by doing more repetitions or more sets of the same exercise, or by combining a high-intensity cardio type exercise with a lower intensity exercise.

The following groups of exercises should take no more than 30 minutes even with a short warmup and cool-down of static stretches at the end.

An example might be doing **Jumping Jacks** for 30 seconds followed by **Crunches** for 60 seconds; you can do this for a total of 5 minutes.

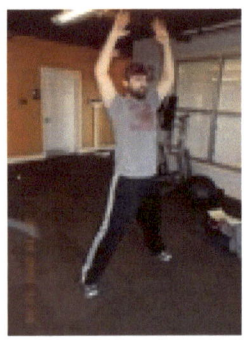
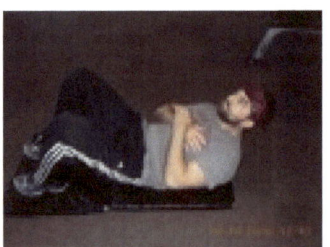

Another example might be to do **Step-ups** on the bed or stairs for 30 seconds followed by slow **Prayer Squats** for 60 seconds. You can do this combination for 5 minutes.

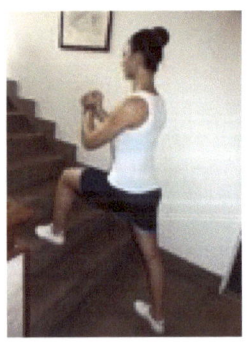
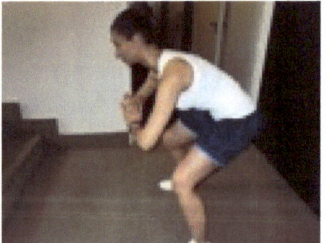

A third example could be doing **Elevated Push-ups** for 30 seconds followed by **Double Crunches** (bring your knees up at the same time your shoulders come off the floor) for 60 seconds. Do this for another 5 minutes.

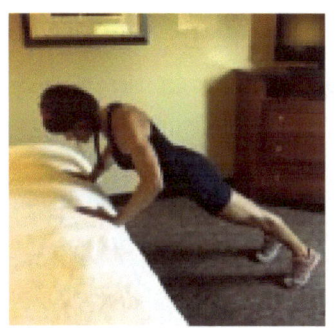 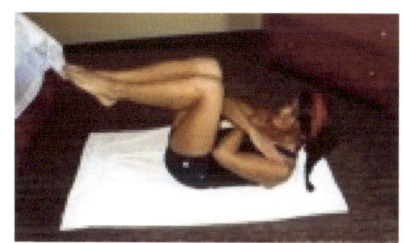

A final example could be **Step Jogging** in the hotel for 1 minute, followed by 2 minutes of walking the halls. You can do this for another 6 minutes, finishing up with a cool-down of **Static Stretches** for a short routine that will keep your body toned while burning that unwanted fat.

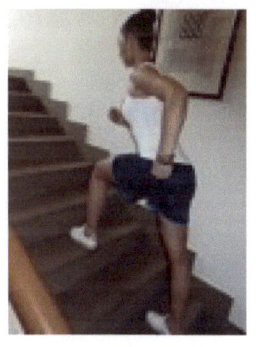 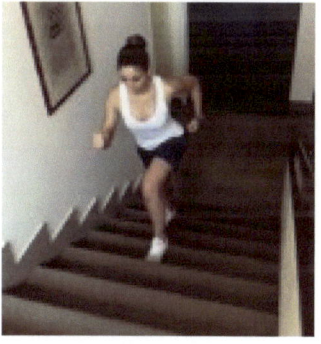

Remember that eating a little snack, preferably low glycemic, a 1/2 hour before the workout will increase your endurance while slowing down your appetite.

Chapter Seven

Step Routine

Every hotel and some multi-story motels have steps that can be used for a great workout. Begin by locating the steps, which could be inside or outside depending on the building; some might be labeled an emergency exit on the inside of the building. Just remember to check the door before you close it to see if it locks from the inside.

You might walk down the steps and run or jog up, saving your knees from the excessive weight that occurs when you apply pressure on the down step.

You can combine step jogging or running with body weight exercises such as Push-ups, Jumping Jacks, Squats, etc.

This routine should take no more than 30 minutes including the Static Stretches at the end:

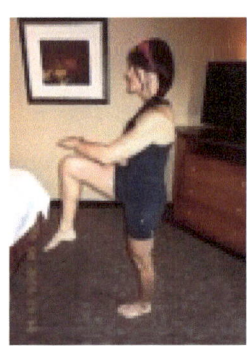

I. **Warm-up**

- Do a slow, high step (march) down the hall.

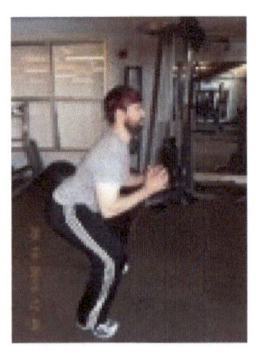

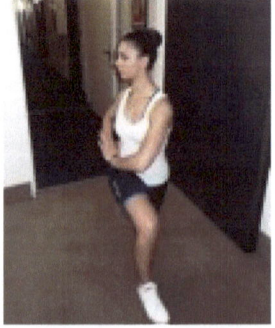

- Come back up the hall doing a lunge and twist.

- Shuffle sideways down the hall and return.

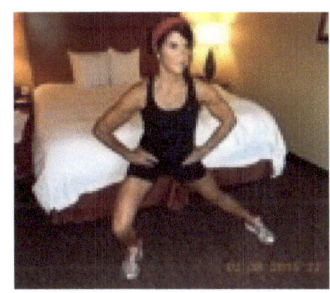

- Do Side Lunges, alternating sides, for 12 reps

- Do 15 Prayer Squats

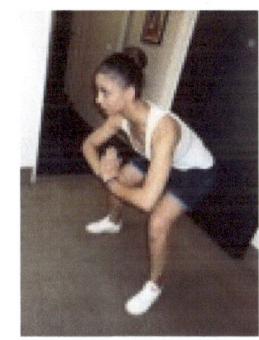

II.   **Step Workout**

- Walk down a flight of stairs, stop at the bottom and do
15 push-ups, using the 3rd or 4th step for your hand placement. Run or jog
back to the top.

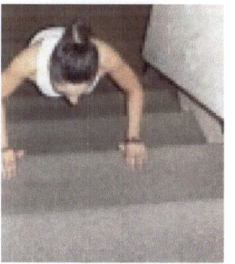

- Walk down to the bottom; this time do 15 jumping jacks; run or jog
back up.

- Walk down again and do Mountain Climbers for 15 seconds and run/jog back up.

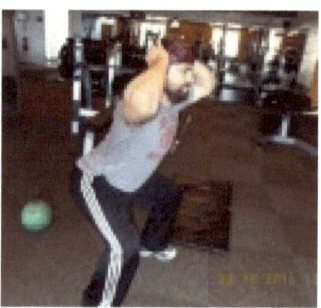

- Walk down again and do 15 Prisoner Squats before running/jogging back up.

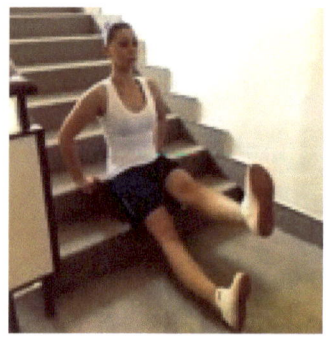

-Walk down again and do 15 Tricep Dips and then return to the top of the stairs.

Repeat the previous five sets of exercises two more times. Remember to rest 60 seconds between each 5-set period. Unless you need to, there should be no rest during the 5 sets of exercises.

This step workout can also be done as a progression routine for an alternative.

An example: Walk down a flight of steps, do 1 push-up, run/jog back up, walk down and do 2 push-ups. Repeat until you get to 10 push-ups. Rest 1 minute and continue with another exercise such as Prisoner Squats.

This is a great way to work on your endurance and strength at the same time.

III. **Static Stretch**

-Below are samples of Static Stretches and some have already been discussed.

Achilles   Hamstring Stretch   Cobra

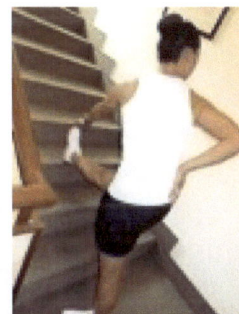 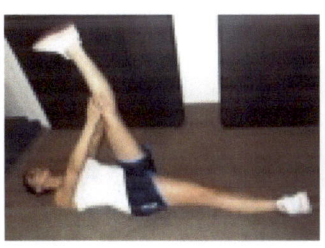 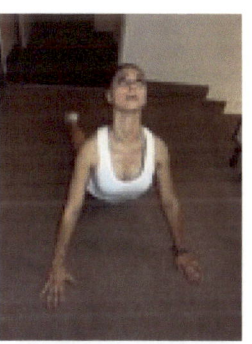

Downward Dog   Cat   Cow

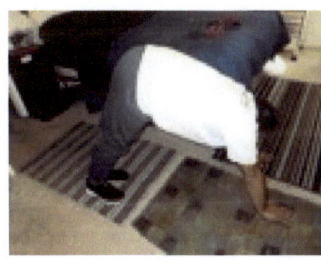 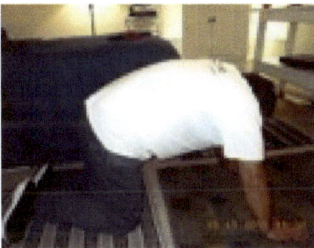 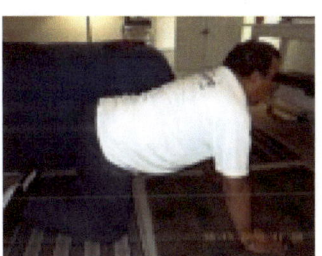

Butter Fly

Low Back Stretch

Pec Stretch

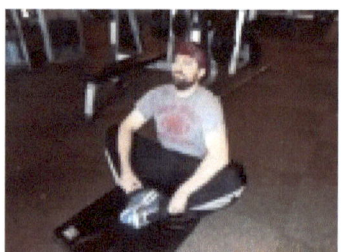
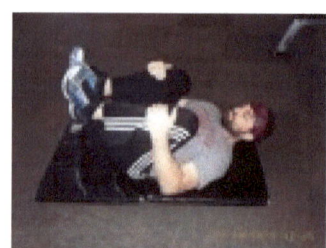
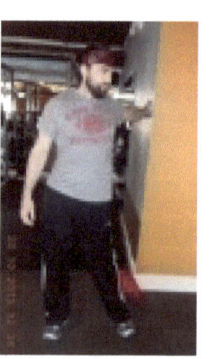

Torso Stretch

Piriformis Stretch

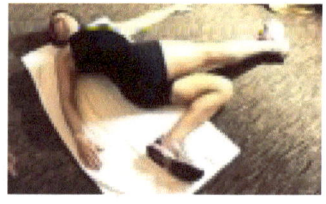
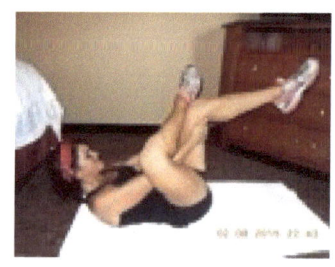
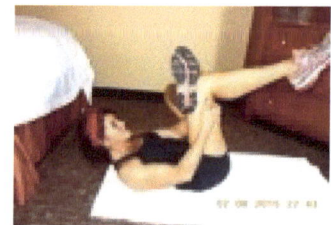

Chapter Eight

Core Only Routine

Many people talk about **core**, but what exactly are they referring to? The core consist of that area of the body from the neck to the hips. We use the muscles of the trunk (e.g. abdominals, obliques, *erector spinae,* muscles along the spine, to create core stability prior to moving into and holding poses for greater strength. Core strength is also good for balance and prevention of low back pain. Most professional golfers have great core strength.

This is a great routine, especially if you want something quick or if you want to combine your evening walk with a workout. Remember that the core has a stabilizing effect on all your muscle groups and i**s probably the most important group of muscles you can work on other than the heart.**

If you take that evening walk, you can use it as the warm-up. Otherwise, follow the Dynamic Stretch routine that we covered earlier. Actually, several High Knees, a dozen Prayer Squats, and 20 Jumping Jacks will suffice for a warm-up for this core routine.

I. **Higher Intensity:**

1/2 Burpee with a Twist Place both hands on the floor in front of you while you shoot your legs out behind; bring your legs back under you and pop up while twisting in the air. Do 1 set of 8 reps.

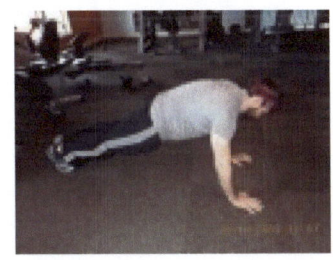 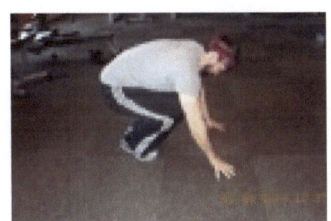 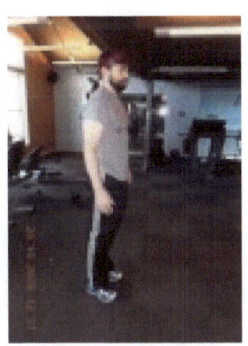

Walk-out Plank From a standing position, reach down and hand crawl out to a Push-up position, hold for 5 to 10 seconds and reverse back to a standing position. Repeat 8 times.

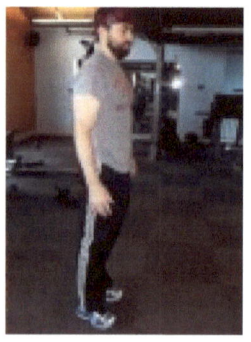

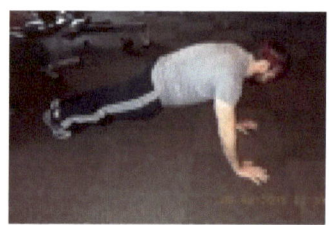

Moguls With hands and body in a Push-up position (feet together), jump with both feet from side to middle to side. Count to 20.

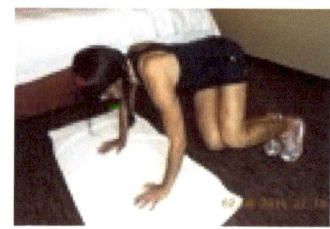

Up and Down Plank Start in a Push-up position, then from your hands, go to your forearms, then back up to your hands. Repeat 8 times. Remember to keep your back and hips in a level position (no butt up in the air).

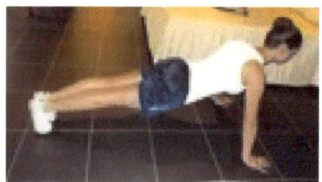

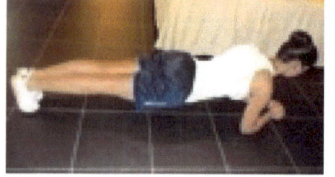

Push-up with Knee to Elbow On the up stage of the Push-up, stop and bring your right knee up to your elbow, then go back down and repeat on the other side. Do 10 reps.

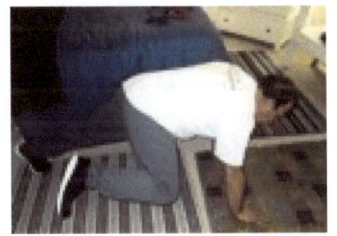 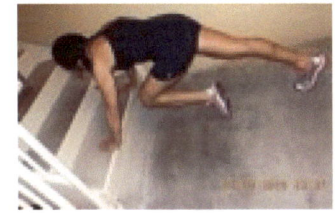

II. Lower Intensity:

Double Crunch   Lying on your back with your arms across your chest and your feet towards the floor with knees bent, bring your knees up towards your chest and bring your shoulders off the floor, then back down. Do 12 reps.

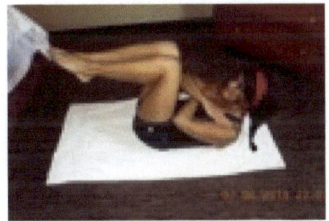

Bird Dog   While on your hands and knees with your back flat as a table top, raise your arm straight out as well as your opposite leg, then repeat on the other side. Hold each pose for 5 seconds and count to 20.

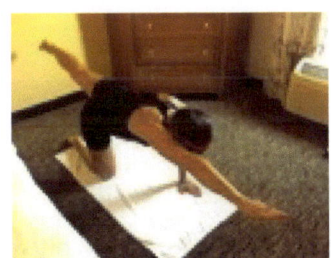

Superman   While lying on your stomach in a prone position with arms outstretched, bring both arms up and both legs up at the same time, hold for 5 seconds, go back down and repeat. Do 10 reps.

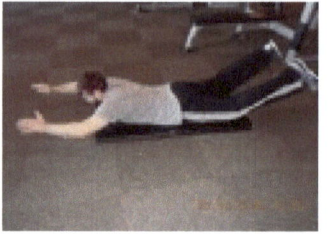

Bridge   While in a supine position, bring your hips up so there is a straight line from your knees to your shoulders.   Lift your leg straight up so that it is level with the opposite knee, then repeat with the opposite leg (hold for 3 seconds). Do 10 reps on each side.

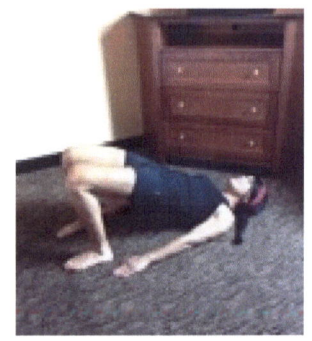

Bridge (Progression)

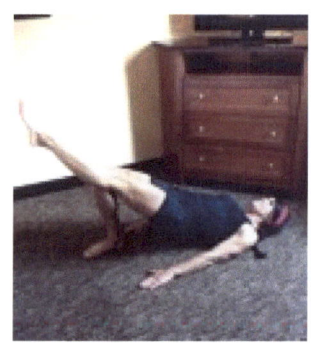

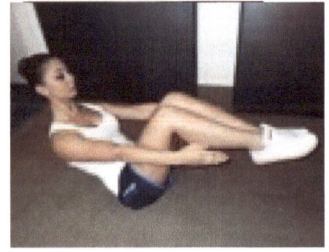

V-Sit While in a seated position, lean back with knees up and feet off the floor and arms out to the side of your legs. Hold for 60 seconds (that's your goal).

III. **Stretch**: Use the Static Stretch techniques we discussed earlier. Spend at least 5 minutes doing your stretches.

This routine should last about 25 to 30 minutes, depending on how much rest you take between each exercise or set. If you have time and want to do more, just go through the routine twice or do 2 sets of each exercise.

Now go out to dinner and enjoy the rest of the evening.

Chapter Nine

Workout with Bands for Strength

Band Workout:

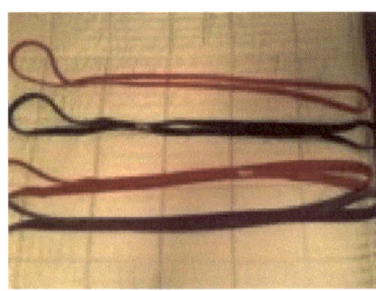 Bands come in varying strengths, usually depicted by color and width. They are normally about 1/8 to 1/4 inch thick and anywhere from 1/2 to 2 inches wide. Of course, the wider and thicker they are, the stronger you need to be in order to use them properly.

Most folks use a 1/8 inch thickness and anywhere from a 1/2 to a 1 inch-width band. You may use two different bands during a session, depending on the particular exercise. Remember, bands are easy to carry, whether in your car, luggage or hanging on the wall in your house.

Band workouts are normally less intense, usually in a heart rate of zone 2 (moderate intensity). You can normally complete a band workout in 30 minutes, but it may take longer depending on how much rest you take between sets. I recommend 10 to 15 seconds rest between sets.

I. Warm-Up

You should always start an exercise routine with a warm-up. There are many ways to warm up your body, and you may have better ones than I do. However, I feel that warming up the main muscle groups is the most efficient way to start. Three or four of these exercises might be sufficient to get the blood moving and the muscles warm. Five to ten minutes is usually adequate.

We will start by doing Squats. Just remember to hinge those hips (push your hips back) and keep that back straight as you go down; never allow the knees to go over the toes (15 reps).

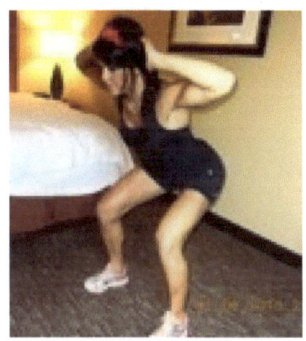 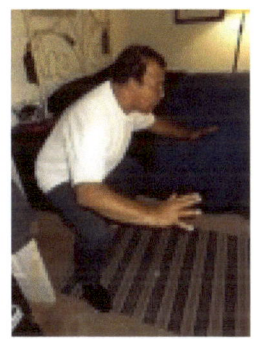 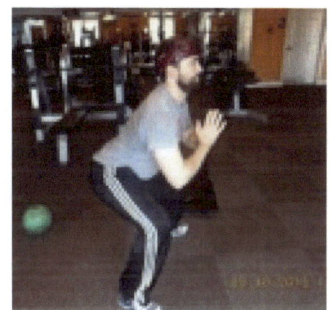

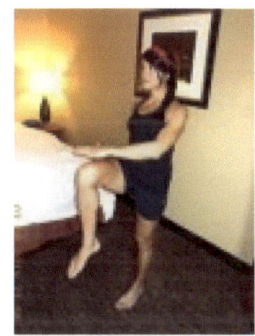

High Knees are next; you can walk or run in place; just keep the knees high (30 seconds) .

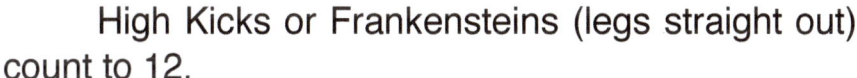

High Kicks or Frankensteins (legs straight out), count to 12.

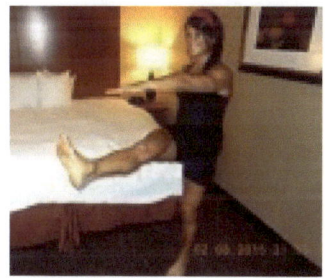

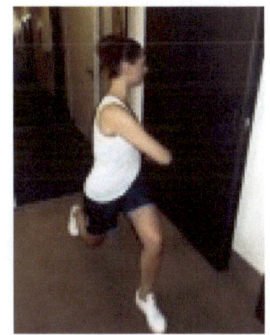

Lunge with a twist, alternate legs and twist to the side of the extended leg, count to 12.

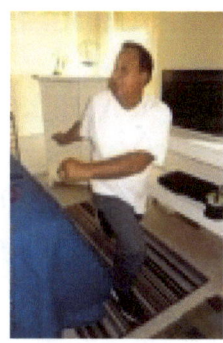

Push-ups - do 12. If modification is necessary, do Push-ups from the knees, the bed or wall Push-ups (lean in with hands against the wall).

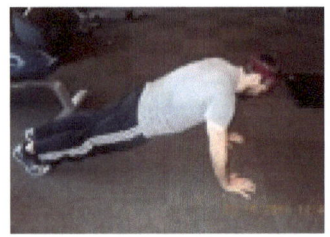 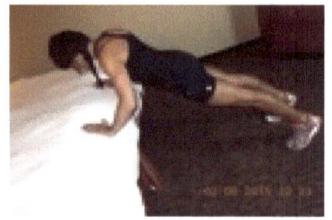 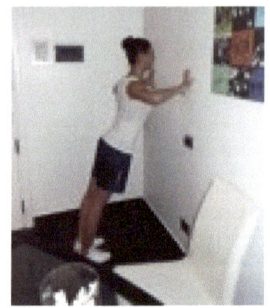

Jumping Jacks, count to 12

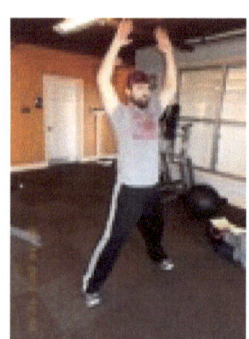 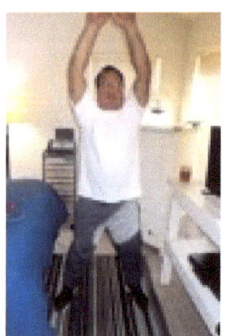

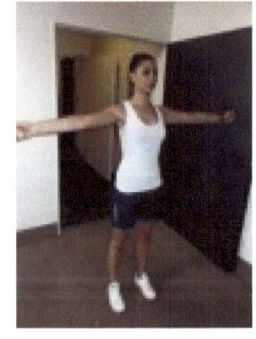

Finally, rotate the arms; with arms straight out, roll frontwards 10 times and backwards 10 times.

II. Upper Body

Chest Flies: Hold the band (doubled up) between your hands and pull the band apart, keeping your arms straight. The closer your hands are, the more strength you'll need to pull the band apart. Try lunging at the same time you stretch the band; this will increase your heart rate. Do 2 sets of 12 to 15 reps.

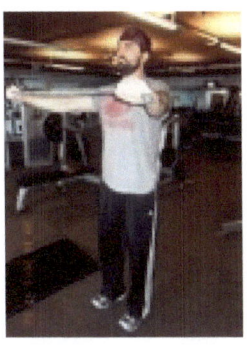 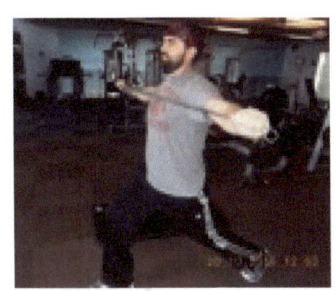 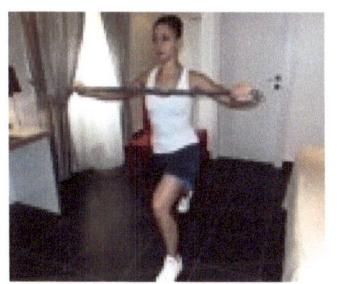

Chest Press: Put the band behind your back, doubled up with your hands on the inside of the band; now press straight out in front of you. Do 2 sets of 12 to 15 reps.

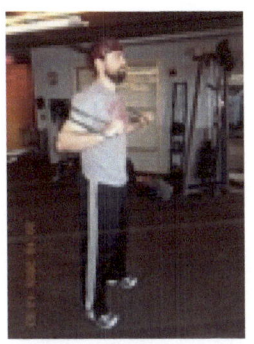 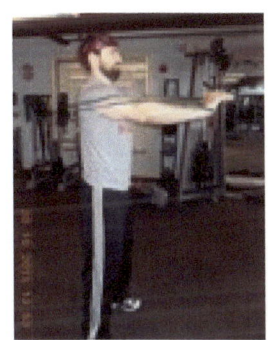 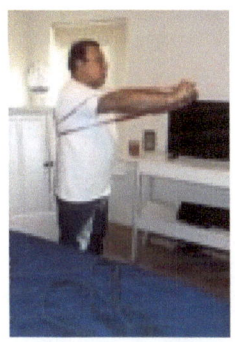

Bent-over Rows: Double up the band under your feet and while bending over at the waist, reach down while grabbing the band with both hands, pull straight up while maintaining a bent-over position; your knees may stay bent at this point. Do 2 sets of 12 to 15 reps.

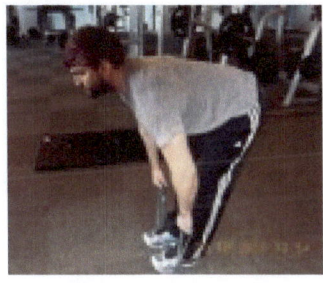 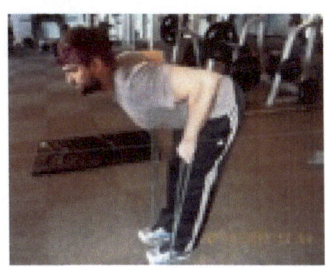 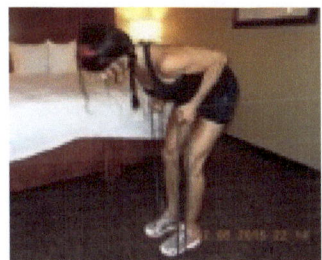

Arm Curls: Place the band under your feet with your hands over the upper portion of the band, and in a standing position, curl up to your chest and bring your arms all the way down to your side. Repeat for 12 to 15 reps. Do 2 sets.

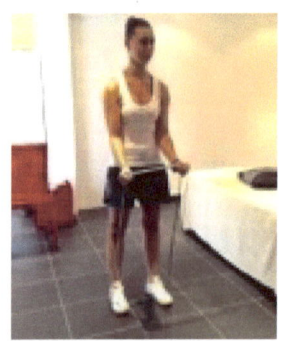 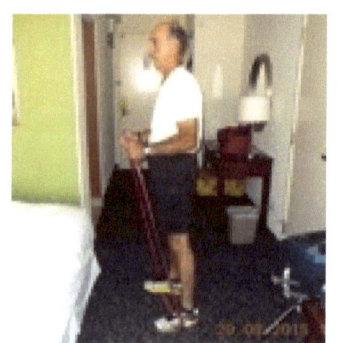 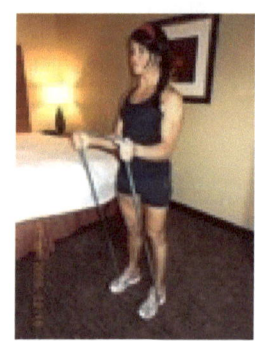

Tricep Extensions: Lying on your back, put the doubled-up band behind your back and with your hands inside the loop of the band, push straight out with your hands together, forming a diamond pattern. Do 2 sets of 12 to 15. You can also stand up doing an overhead Tricep Extension.

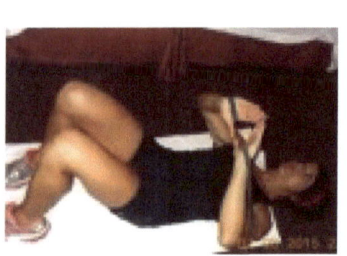 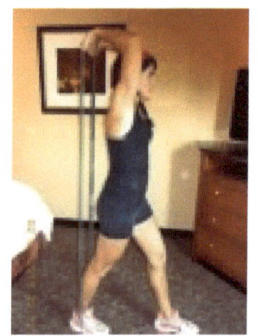 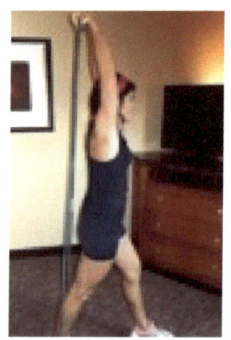

Seated rows: Seating on the floor, put the doubled-up band under your feet. With the band in both hands and seated in an upright position, pull the band to your chest with your palms down. Do 2 sets of 12 to 15 reps.

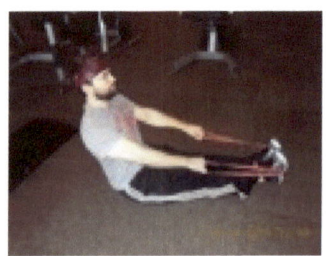 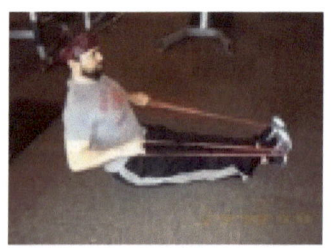 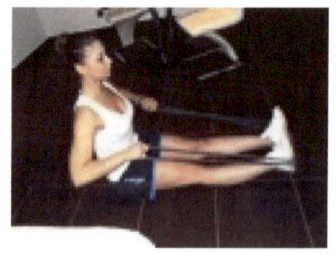

Shoulder Raises: In a standing position with part of the band under your feet and the other part in your hands, palms down, pull the band up under your chin. Do 2 sets of 12 to 15 reps.   If your want stronger resistance, spread your feet farther apart before pulling the band up.

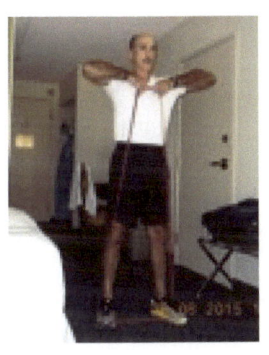
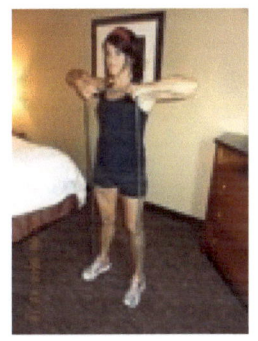

III. **Lower Body**

Squats: Place part of the band under your feet and lift the other half up to your shoulders, holding on with both hands. Now squat down, keeping your back straight and pushing your hips back. Do 2 sets of 15.

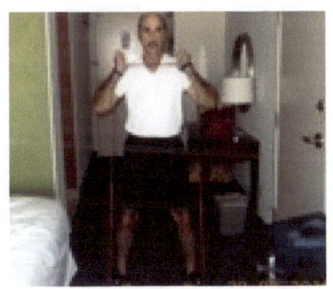
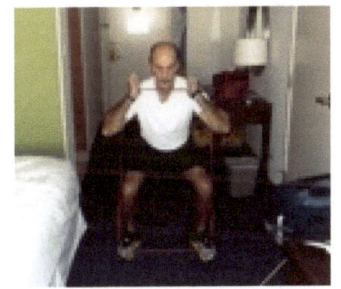
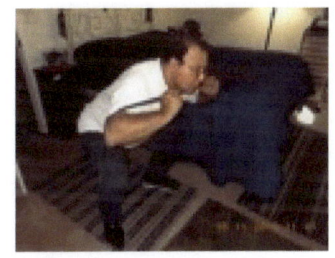

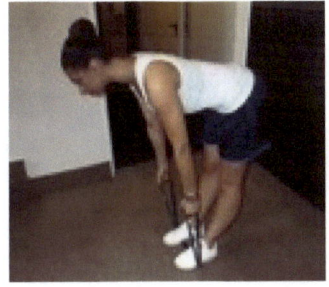
Romanian Dead Lifts (RDLs): Place the band doubled over under your feet, keeping your legs fairly straight; bend over at the waist and with both hands pull the band up as you straighten your body in a standing position. Do 2 sets of 12 to 15
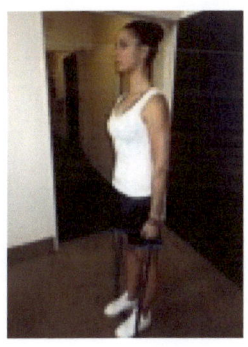

Side Lunges: Place part of the band under your feet and cross the upper part of the band with your hands. Standing with feet shoulder width apart, extend your left leg out to the side, keeping your toes pointed straight ahead. Now bring it back to the middle and repeat for 10 reps, then do the same thing to the right leg. Do 2 sets.

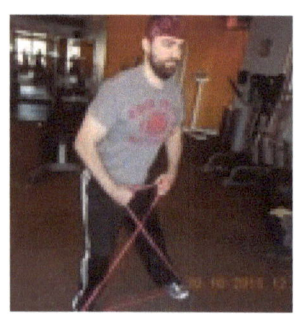

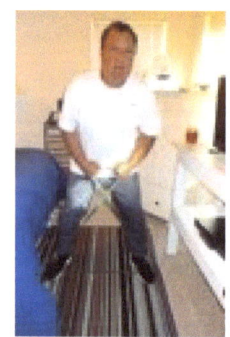

Posterior (Backward) Lunge: Place part of the band under your right foot and lift the other end up to your shoulders, holding with both hands. Now step back with your left leg (Posterior Lunge) into a backward lunge and stand, repeat 10 times; do the same for the right leg, putting the band under your left foot.

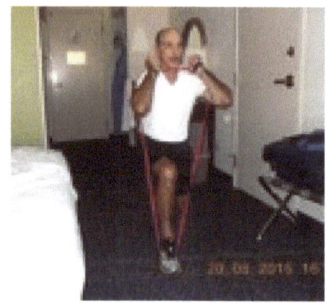

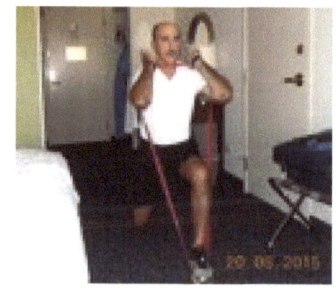

Stretch: Here again, do your Static Stretches (no bouncing). Hold each stretch for 15 to 30 seconds. With your elbows flared out to the sides, stretch back as if to touch the elbows together behind you.

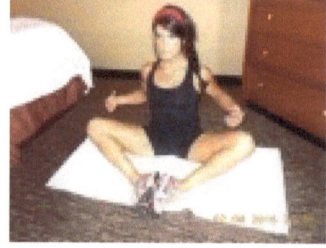

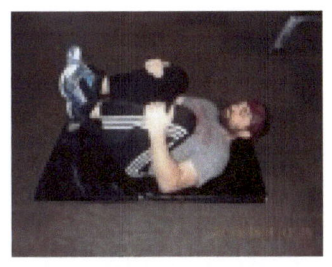

Next, lie flat and bring your knees to your chest, and hold.

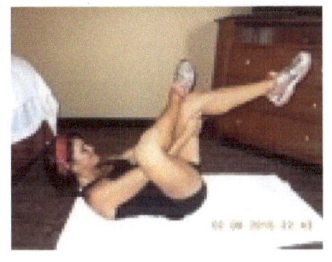

Bring your feet down flat on the floor and cross your right ankle over the left knee; grab behind the knee and pull toward you; hold, switch sides.

Stretch your right leg straight out flat on the floor and bring your left leg straight up preferably at a 90-degree angle; grab the back of your calf or thigh and pull gently towards you, hold, then switch legs.

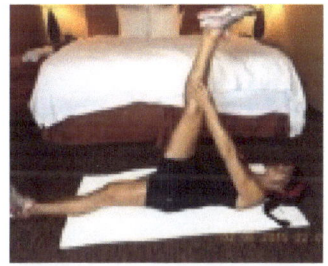

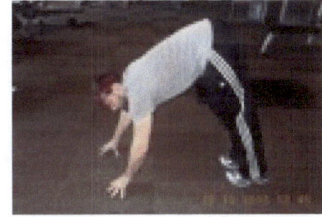

Next go to all fours, feet and hands and do the yoga move called Downward Dog. This will stretch your Achilles and calf muscles.

Go from here down to hands and knees and do the yoga Cat position followed by the Cow, hold for 10 sec.; finally, go to a prone position with your hands under the shoulders and push upward to the yoga Cobra position.

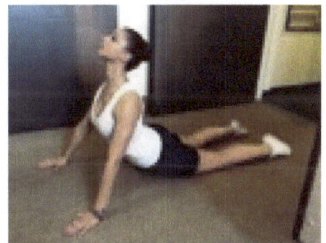

I would suggest doing the Band Workout when you get back to your room after the day's business meetings or activities. This way, you won't have to hurry and you can eat a leisurely dinner afterwards.

Chapter Ten

5X6s Routine (Rest-Based)

This routine incorporates circuit training consisting of 6 different groups of exercises, 5 minutes continuously for each group (1 min. rest between groups). When doing **rest-based exercises**, you decide when to rest and for how long during the 5-minute session. The idea is to go all out doing an exercise until you feel that you can't give it all you have; then rest until you feel you can give it a 100% again, then start where you left off.

Follow the warm-up (Dynamic Stretches) I discussed in the previous chapters.

Circuit

1a. Prayer Squats/Prisoner Squats (12 count)

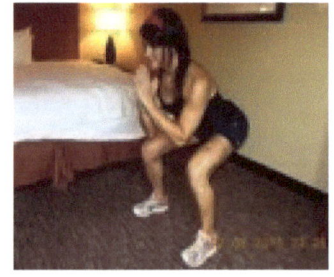 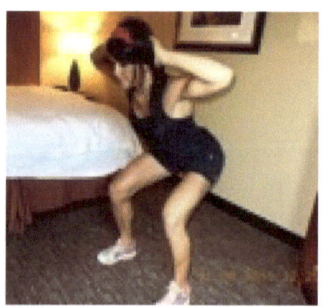

1b. Push-ups (12 count)

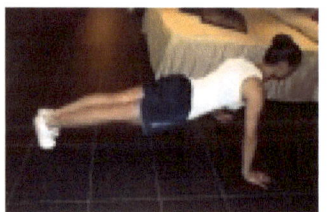

1c. Steam engine (12 count)

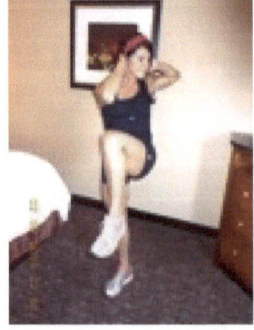 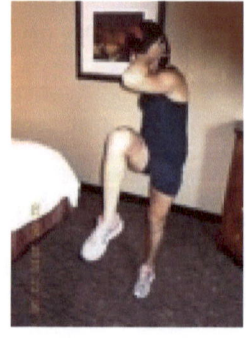

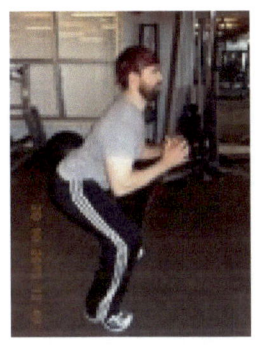 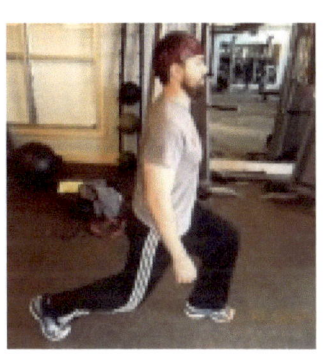

2a. Squat and Lunge (alternate legs - 12 count)

2b. Mountain Climbers (12 count)

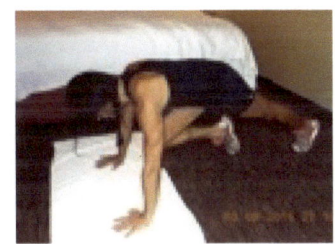

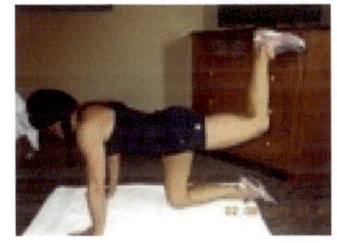

2c. Donkey Kicks (12 reps for each leg)

3a. Jumping Jacks (12 count)

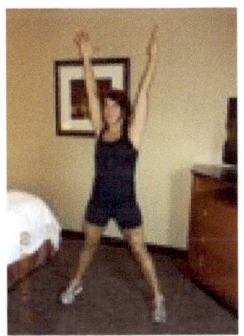 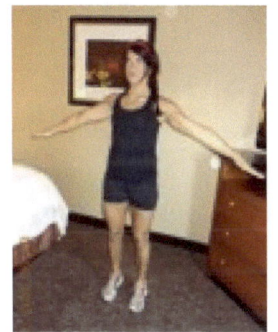

3b. One Leg RDL with Reach (do 12 on each leg)

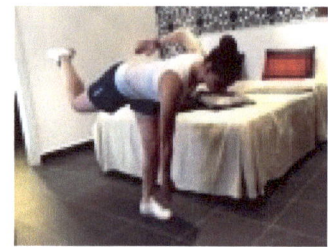 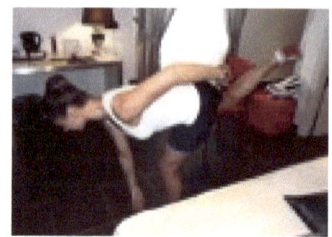

3c. Crunches (4 sec. count) do 12

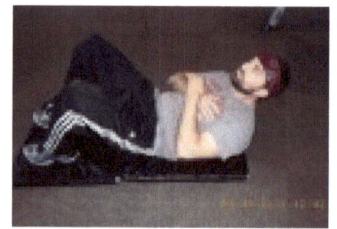

4a. Frog Squats (stay in a
   squat position through
   the exercise - 12 count)

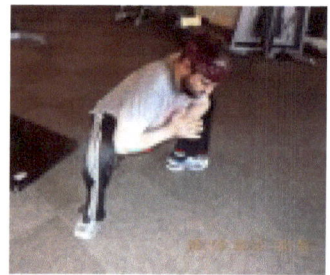 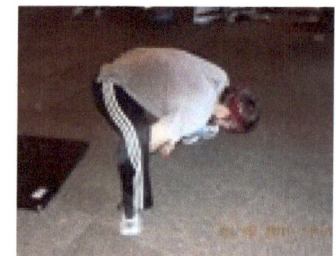

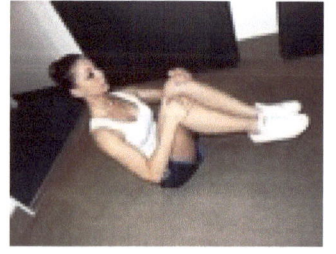 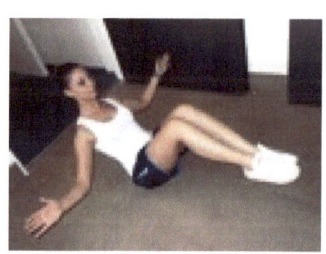   4b. Ab Flies (12 count)

4c. Moguls (feet together,
jump side to back to
opposite side - 12 count)

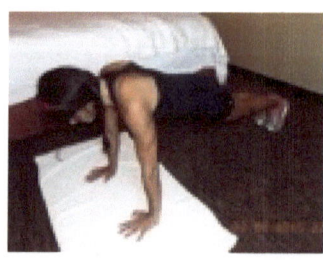 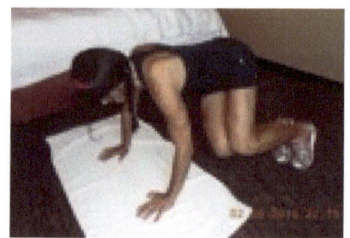

5a. 1/2 Burpee (minus the Push-up - 12 count)

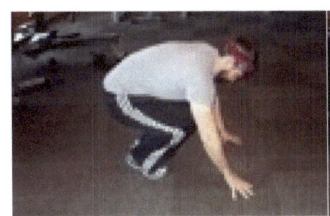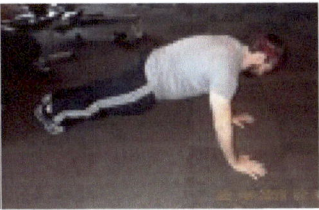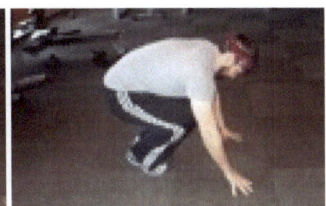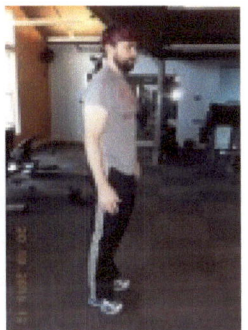

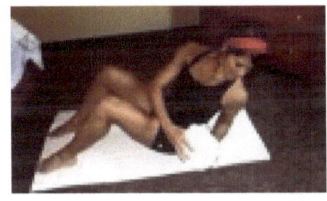

5b. Russian Twist (feet up for more progression; twist side to side - 12 count)

5c. Frog Jumps (point toes out, jump forward and walk back - 12 count)

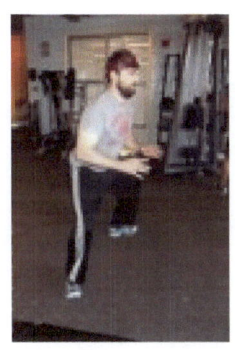

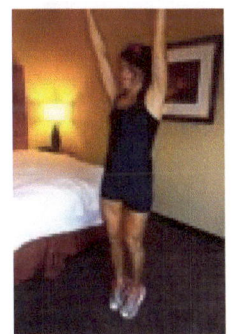

6a. Power Squats or Jump Squats (12 count)

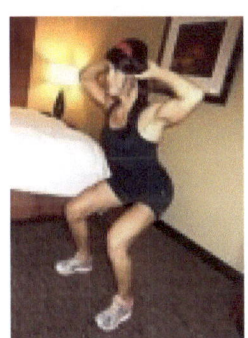

6b. Plank (can also be done from the knees - 12 second count)

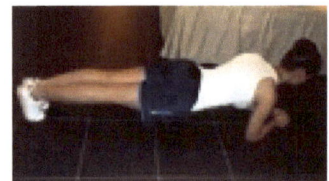 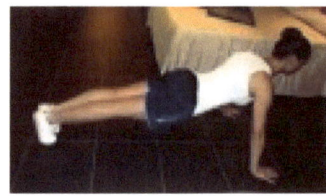

6c. Legs to the Sky and Reach
(keep legs straight as you reach -
Count to 12)

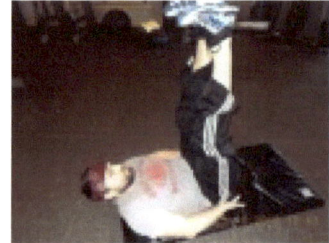

Static Stretch: Refer to previous chapters for muscle group stretches. Don't forget that stretching is an important part of your workouts. It provides a cool-down period, lengthens the muscles and prevents tightening of the muscles that can cause pain and stiffness.

This routine should take about 45 minutes including warm-up and stretching. It is a great routine when you get back to your room after work or meetings. **Don't forget - even if you work from home, this program is a great way to stay in shape.**

Chapter Eleven

5-Day Program

I have given you several routines to follow, but now I want to give you a 5-day program to follow for that entire week on the road in your Hotel/ Motel. You can also use this program for a possible second week, or if you're staying for a longer period, you can vary the order of the exercises and change the intensity or duration to make it a little more challenging.

Day I

Morning: If possible, get that **30-minute walk or jog/run** in before breakfast. This will wake you up and feeling fresh for that first meeting.

Evening: If you're a beginner, start off slowly and use the recommended routine in Chapter 3, **The Beginner's Workout.** Otherwise, if you're carrying exercise bands, the **Band Workout** (Ch. 9) is ideal for the first evening or you can do the **Body Weight 30X30** (Ch. 4) exercises. Remember to get a small snack in 30 to 45 minutes prior to the workout.

Day 2

Morning: This could be a good day to try the **Step Workout** from Chapter 7. You're up early, so the halls and steps of the hotel/motel shouldn't be too busy. You might not have a lot of time, so do a quick warm-up and try the **Progression Routine** also mentioned in Chapter 7, with push-ups.

Evening: This is a good time for that **30-minute walk** again. Of course, this depends on the weather. If things are bad outside, re-do the **step routine**, using the **Progression**. Don't forget to stretch after any workout.

Day 3

Morning: This might be a good time to do the Core-Only Routine. After the warm-up, do 1 set of each exercise as suggested in Chapter 8. This should allow you to go eat that big breakfast before work.

Evening: This is a good time to use the exercise bands again and follow the **Band Routine** in Chapter 9. If bands are not available, or if you desire a more intense workout, the **Metabolic Workout** in Chapter 6 is a great change-up. This should wear you out, so after dinner, the sheets might be your best bet.

Day 4

Morning: It's time for that **morning walk, jog/run** again, but make sure you hydrate. Drink water before you start. Even if you don't have a full 30 minutes to devote, 15 or 20 minutes will do. Now shower and eat breakfast before the work day.

Evening: This is a good time to push yourself a little harder, so I'm suggesting the **5X6s Routine** from Chapter 10. It will take about 45 minutes, so allow some time before you go out for that high-protein meal you want to eat.

Day 5

Morning: This is usually the day when you pack up for the trip home in the afternoon, so I suggest just doing a **15 minute walk/jog** for a warm-up and finishing with some of the **Dirty Dozen** exercises from Chapter 5 for another 15 minutes. You can concentrate on the **Core Exercises** and throw in some cardio/strength moves to work up a sweat.

Remember, you can modify any of the exercises to fit your level of fitness. As you get used to doing the different routines, you will find yourself increasing the intensity either by doing more repetitions, shortening the rest periods between reps or by increasing the time you spend working out.

The 5-day program can be used every time you're away on the road or at your house. To keep from getting bored or in a rut, all you need to do is incorporate a different routine daily, change the order of the routine, or change the intensity of each exercise. If you're away from home for a week or a month, this program will give you all the exercises needed to keep you feeling healthy and your body in shape

Summary

In summing up the concept of my Hotel/Motel workout plan, I would like to reemphasize that it is derived from my exercise experiences while traveling, working at the YMCA and doing in-home training. The main issue I see with clients is that they have very little time to exercise on a regular basis. Between work and caring for children or taking out the dog, they tend to put exercising on the back burner, and only make time for a regular routine when they are desperate to lose weight or get into shape for a sporting event.

So basically, I wrote this book to help people find the time and type of routine that will help them stay in shape, maintain good health, and get them ready for any activity they desire to do.

You can do the Hotel/Motel Work-out when you're on the road or at home; it is quick and simple. There is plenty of time for work and family.

Healthy living should be the goal for all of us, because we need to stay healthier longer in our lives so we can enjoy our families, take part in community activities and feel better as we get older. Staying away from the the doctor's office is also a perk of staying healthy.

Remember that you can use these routines any way you like. If you don't have 30 or 40 minutes to spare one day, you can cut the exercises down to just a few and do 15 or 20 minutes, or if one day you have more time, you can do 45 minutes to an hour. The main thing is to do some type of rigorous movement/exercise 4 to 5 days per week. I always say to my wife, " Break a sweat! " Then you know you've accomplished your exercise goal for that day.

Be in charge of your life and know that it's never too late to start an exercise program. It will mentally and physically energize you and greatly enhance your self-esteem.

For any questions concerning the exercises in this book, you may contact the author at
vpane46@gmail.com